Let's Discover the South Beach Diet Together

This Cookbook Will Give You Awesome and Delicious Recipes to Stay Lean!

BY

Rachael Rayner

License Notes

No part of this Book can be reproduced in any form or by any means including print, electronic, scanning or photocopying unless prior permission is granted by the author.

All ideas, suggestions and guidelines mentioned here are written for informative purposes. While the author has taken every possible step to ensure accuracy, all readers are advised to follow information at their own risk. The author cannot be held responsible for personal and/or commercial damages in case of misinterpreting and misunderstanding any part of this Book

Table of Contents

Introduction

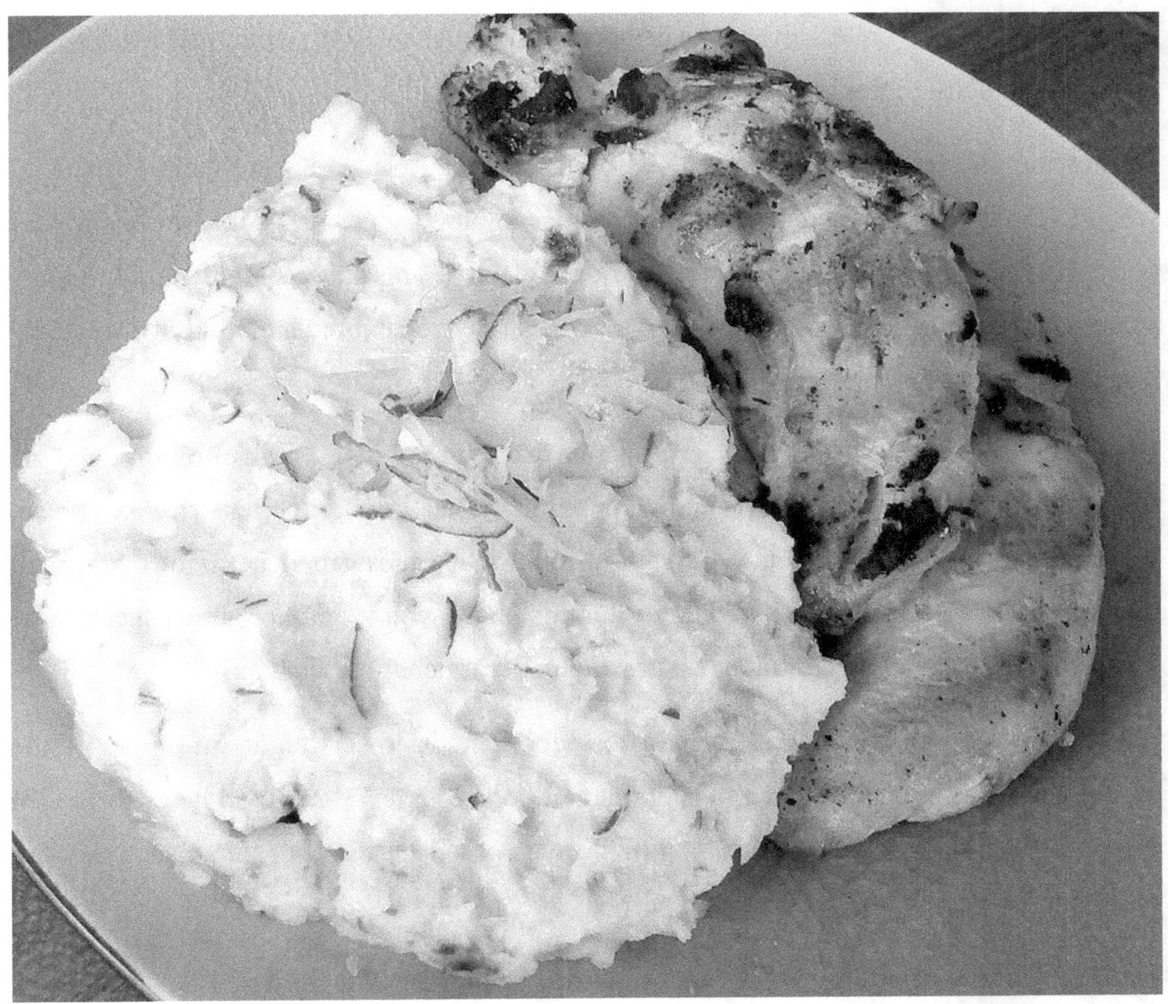

The south beach diet, in a nutshell, consists in 3 phases. During the first 2 weeks, you will get rid of the starchy foods such as potatoes, rice, pasta, fruits, and alcohol. Basically, you will eliminate any high sugary or carbs food items from your diet. Black tea, black coffee, and water will be your beverages of choice.

You should avoid any processed foods or the ones you can't tell exactly what they are made of, even by reading the list of ingredients on the labels. You can eat nuts and most cheeses and lean meats, so you will get plenty of proteins, don't you worry. This is not a dangerous diet to start; however, as always, we recommend you speak to your preferred health professional before jumping into this dieting adventure.

During the first stage of the diet, you should expect to lose a significant amount of weight. Because you will reduce the fluctuations in blood sugar levels in your body, your body will start adjusting to the new foods you will feed it. This phase should include mainly some fish, lean meat, chicken, turkey, eggs, non-starchy vegetables, and low-fat cheese and dairy products in moderation.

During the second phase, starting at your third week of the diet, you can reintroduce the fresh fruits, some types of cereals and whole grains pasta or whole grains rice and bread. However, for grains and fruits, you should reintroduce these food items in very small quantities. Don't be disappointed that during this phase, you might not notice such a high weight loss. You should continue losing weight, but much more gradually.

Actually, some individuals with weight loss goals much lower might simply apply the second phase, as they don't need to deprive their body of a few other food items forbidden in phase one. The second phase is allowing you to add a few fun items such as dark chocolate, sweet potatoes, some fresh berries, so enjoy it!

Finally, you will be ready for the longest phase of your diet, the third phase. This means that you can start eating what you want. Well, wait a minute! Some people misunderstand this phase or this truth of life. If you start eating fried foods, processed foods, high sugar drinks, don't get fooled, you will put back the weight you lost and maybe more. So, be smart and do it right.

So, the third phase is basically going back to a long-term lifestyle, dieting wise.

Taco style lettuce wraps

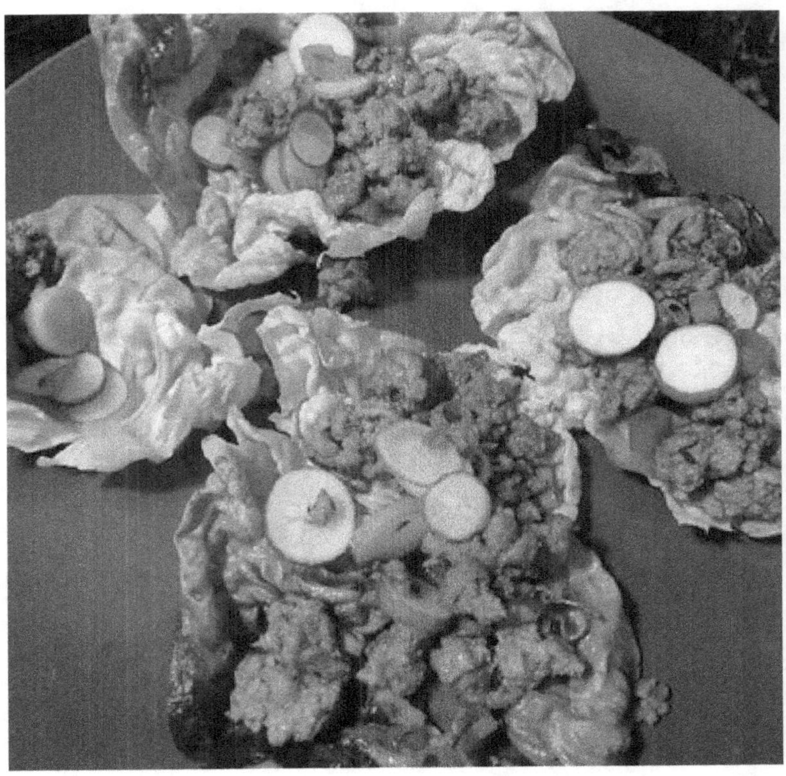

I am sure you have seen this type of wraps on the menu at some of your favorite restaurants. It is a very popular way to add some delicious ingredients together, and instead of using tortillas, breads, or other carb-loaded ingredients, you can simply use lettuce leaves. Romaine lettuce works great for this. The leaves are large and crispy, holding the content of your wrap just fine.

Ingredients:

- 4 large lettuce leaves (romaine lettuce or other of your choice)

- 1-pound lean turkey meat

- ¼ diced red onion

- 1 medium diced fresh tomato

- ½ cup low fat cottage cheese

- 1 Tbsp. olive oil

- Fresh minced cilantro

Servings: 4

Preparation time: 45 minutes

Nutritional information (per serving = 2 lettuce wraps)

Calories: 220

Carbs: 8g

Proteins: 22g

Fats: 15g

Method:

In a large skillet, heat the oil and sautéed the red onion for a few minutes before adding the ground meat.

Cook the meat for about 20 minutes, kept stirring to make sure it stays rumbly.

Meanwhile, prepare the lettuce, plate and add a full tablespoon of cottage cheese in each.

When the meat is fully cooked, add some in each leaf-wrap and sprinkle some fresh tomatoes and fresh chopped cilantro on it.

Awesome chicken stew

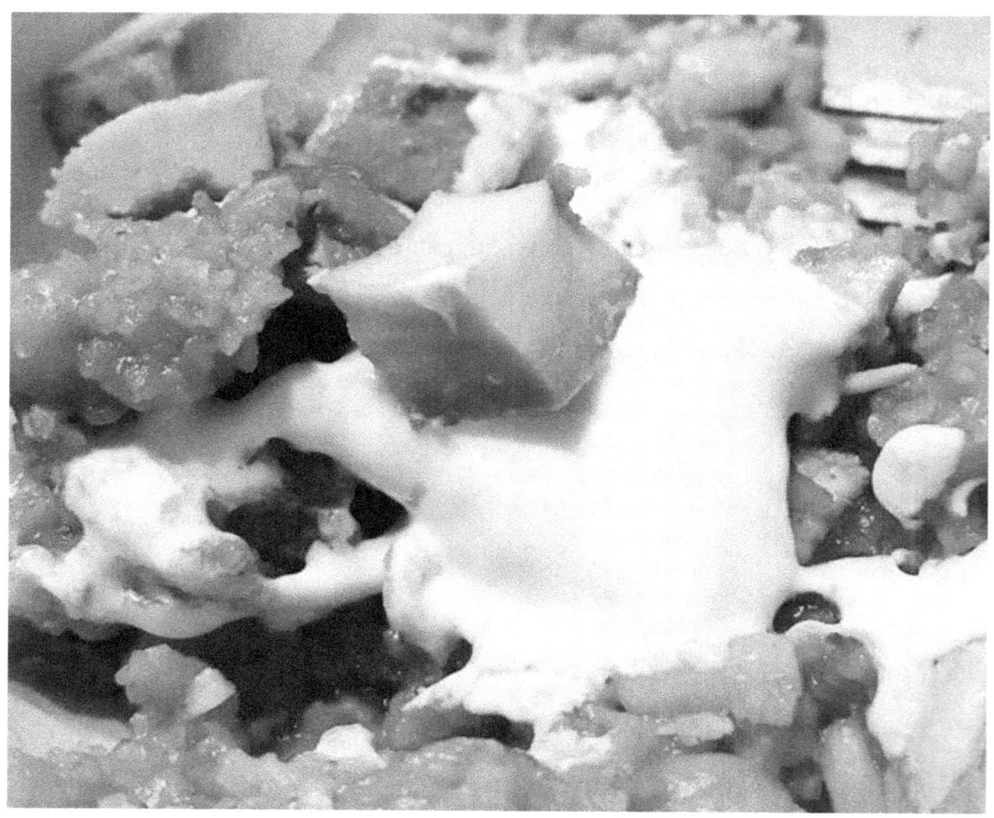

Did you think you had to say goodbye to all the awesome stews, casseroles, soups, or any other yummy warm meals you like to prepare because you are following the south beach diet? Remember, it is in the sauce: the taste and yumminess of the meal, but that's where all these unnecessary calories can hide. For this recipe, we will suggest a great compromise for you.

Ingredients:

- 3 large cooked and shredded chicken breasts

- 1 small chopped yellow onion

- 2 minced garlic cloves

- 1 large can dice tomatoes with chilies

- 1 cup low fat vegetables broth

- 1 tbsp. white balsamic vinegar

- 2 tbsp. agave syrup

- 1 tsp. chili powder

- 1 tsp. red pepper flakes

- 1 Tbsp. lemon juice

- ½ tsp. cumin

- 1 tbsp. olive oil

- Salt, black pepper

Toppings suggestions: diced avocados, light sour cream, low fat shredded sharp cheddar

Servings: 4-6

Preparation time: 60 minutes

Nutritional information (per serving =about 1 ½ cup of stew)

Calories: 299

Carbs: 16g

Proteins: 24g

Fats: 14g

Method:

I always opt to use the crockpot for this recipe, I think it's just easier.

Use chicken you cooked previously and shred it.

In a skillet, heat the oil and cook the garlic and onions for about 5 minutes.

Then in the crockpot, add all the veggies, including the tomatoes, the broth, the cooked chicken, vinegar and all spices.

Stir and set om low temperature for 4 hours.

When you are ready to serve, add some of your favorite toppings as suggested above.

Strawberry Yogurt

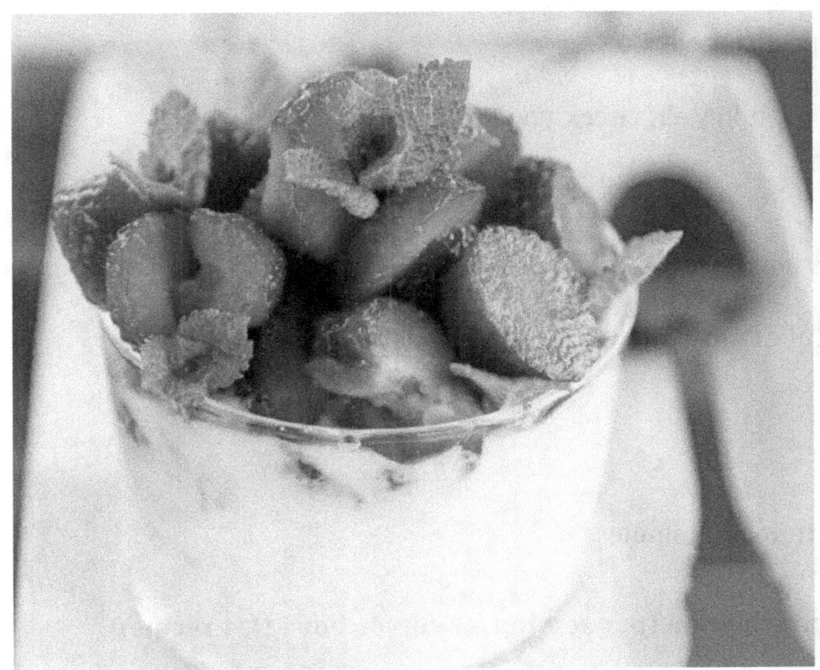

You can choose to prepare and eat this recipe for a quick, satisfying dessert, or as a quick and healthy breakfast. It will be thicker than a shake, so I suggest you eat it with a spoon instead of using a straw.

Ingredients:

- 4 large scoops of vanilla protein shake (low carbs of course)

- 2 Tbsp. chia seeds

- 1 cup plain low-fat Greek yoghurt

- 1 cup fresh raspberries or strawberries your choice

- 3 cups unsweetened coconut milk

- Handful of unsweetened coconut flakes as topping

Servings: 3-4

Preparation time: 20 minutes

Nutritional information (per serving =1 cup or bowl (1/4 recipe))

Calories: 160

Carbs: 11g

Proteins: 4 g

Fats: 4g

Method:

In a large mixing bowl, mix all the ingredients, except the fruits. You could use the blender and blend for just a few seconds, so you can still have some great thickness and consistency. I prefer to simply use a wooden spoon and mix for several minutes.

Pour into 4 individual bowls or cups and divide the fruits as toppings and the coconut flakes.

Delicious baked garlic salmon filets

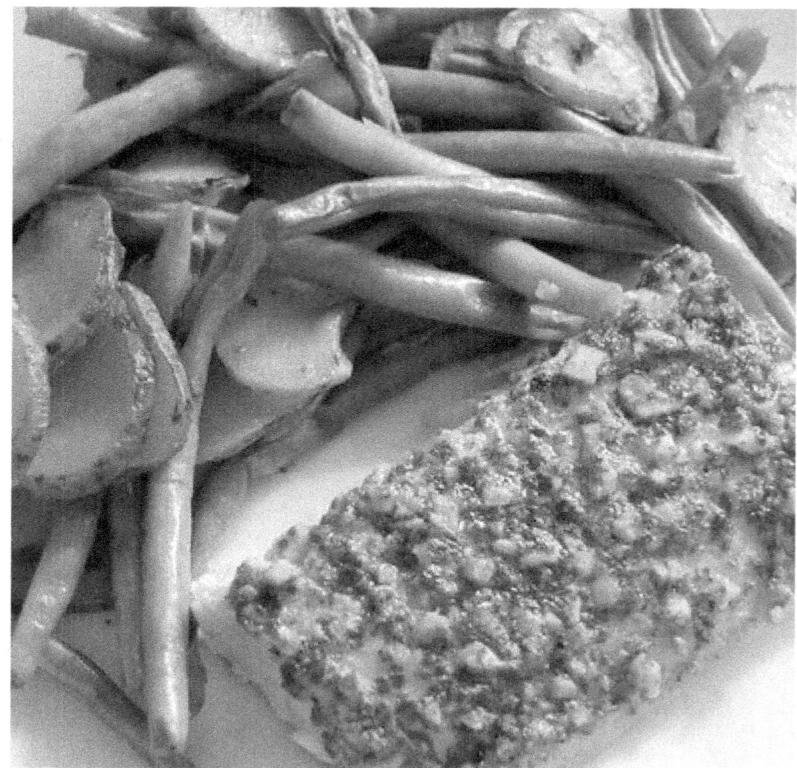

There is no right or wrong way to cook salmon. Salmon is the best fish to eat no matter what diet you are on, in my opinion. It is loaded with omega 3, the good type of fats that you want in your diet, and it is very delicious.

Ingredients:

- 4 salmon filets

- 2 Tbsp. avocado oil

- 2 Tbsp. minced fresh garlic

- Salt, black pepper

- 1 Tbsp. cilantro paste

- ½ cup chopped sundried tomatoes

- 1 cup hot water

- 1 tbsp.., miso pasta

- 1 Tbsp. balsamic vinegar

- Fresh minced parsley to decorate

Servings: 4

Preparation time: 50 minutes

Nutritional information (per serving =1 salmon filet)

Calories: 282

Carbs: 8g

Proteins: 19g

Fats: 21g

Method:

Preheat the oven to 350 degrees F.

Grease a large baking dish and place the filets skin down.

In a medium mixing bowl, combine the miso pasta and the hot water, set aside for now.

In a different bowl, combine the vinegar, garlic, avocado oil, the cilantro paste (you can purchase any store in produce section)

Use a brush to brush off each salmon filets with the oily mixture.

Place the salmon I the oven for 10 minutes.

Remove from the oven and pour the miso pasta mixture on top and sprinkle the chopped sundried tomatoes as well.

Place in the oven for another 10-12 minutes.

When done serve with fresh parsley on top.

Egg muffins

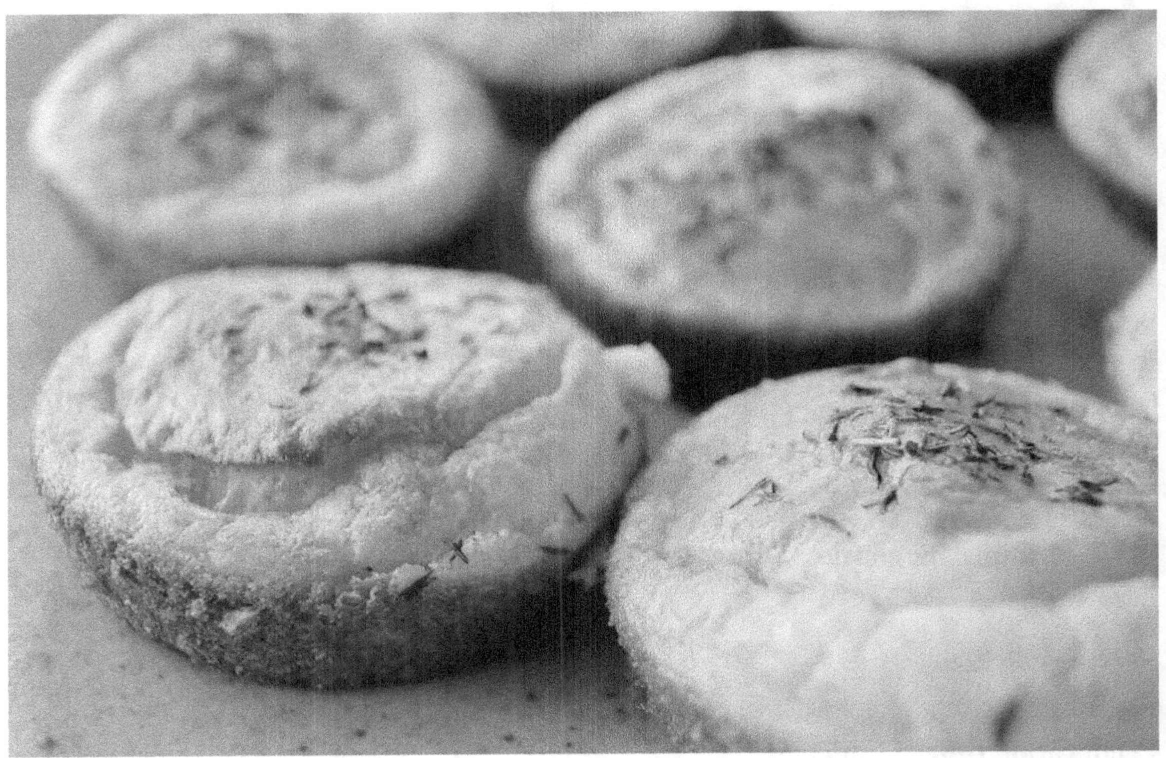

These egg muffins are the perfect on-the-go breakfast or pre-workout snack. They are nutritious, but also so easy to prepare. Just mix all these wonderful ingredients together, bake, and let cool down until they are ready to munch! You can add your favorite veggies in them; we happened to love bell peppers.

Ingredients:

- 8 large eggs

- ½ cup skim milk

- 1 cup low fat ricotta cheese

- ½ diced green bell pepper

- ½ diced red bell pepper

- Salt, black pepper

- ½ tsp. garlic powder

- ½ tsp. onion powder

- 1 tbsp. chili powder

Servings: 8-12

Preparation time: 55 minutes

Nutritional information (per serving =1 muffin)

Calories: 320

Carbs: 16g

Proteins: 22g

Fats: 15g

Method:

Preheat the oven to 350 degrees F.

Grease a muffin tin and set aside.

In a large mixing bowl, combine the eggs, milks, ricotta cheese and all seasonings.

In a medium pan, heat the oil and cook for 5-6 minutes the bell peppers.

Add to the first mixture and then combine.

Pour into the muffin holes and bake for about 45 minutes. Serve as soon as done and cooled down.

Healthy shrimp stir fry

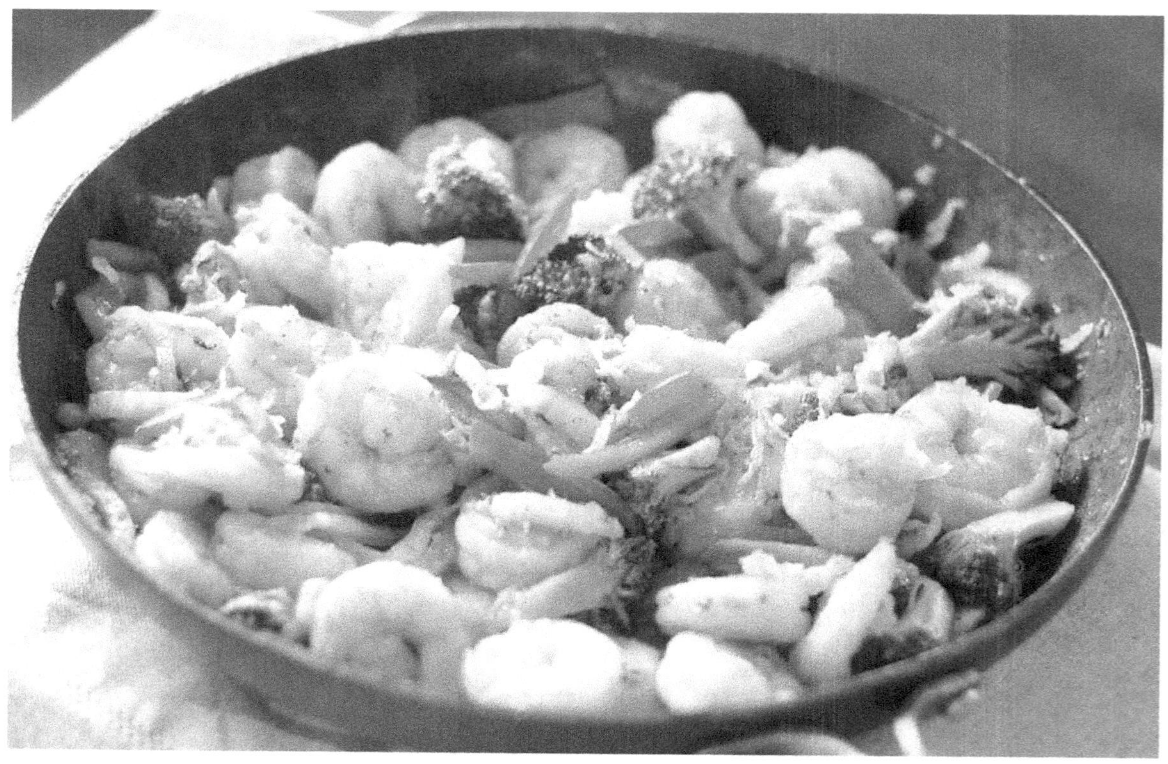

No need to go and order this very heavy and carbs loaded stir fry, from the local Chinese restaurant of your neighborhood. Why don't you learn how to make this delicious stir fry that your whole family will enjoy? We propose using the shrimp as a protein, but you can very well use chicken, beef, or pork for their recipe, and it would be fantastic.

Ingredients:

- 1 pound medium deveined and peeled uncooked shrimp

- 2 cups fresh snap peas

- 2 minced green onion

- 1 large chopped yellow bell pepper

- 2 tbsp. sesame oil

- 1 tbsp. sesame seeds

- 1 Tbsp. fresh minced ginger

- 1 Tbsp. Fresh minced garlic

- 1 Tbsp. red pepper flakes

- 2 cups low fat chicken broth

- Salt, black pepper

- 1 Tbsp. hot sauce

Servings: 3-4

Preparation time: 45 minutes

Nutritional information (per serving = about 1 cup veggies and 6 shrimp)

Calories: 320

Carbs: 16g

Proteins: 21g

Fats: 14g

Method:

Use a wok or a large skillet for this recipe

In a mixing bowl, you should first combine the oil, ginger, garlic hot sauce, salt, pepper and red flakes pepper.

Add the shrimp in the mixture and let them marinade 15 minutes or more.

Meanwhile heat some oil in the pan of your choice and cook the onion, yellow pepper and snap peas 5 minutes before adding the shrimp.

Shrimp should take about 15-20 minutes to be ready on medium heat.

Add the chicken broth as needed to create a lovely sauce.

Serve on a bed of zucchini noodles if you like.

Sprinkle with sesame seeds.

Veggie burger

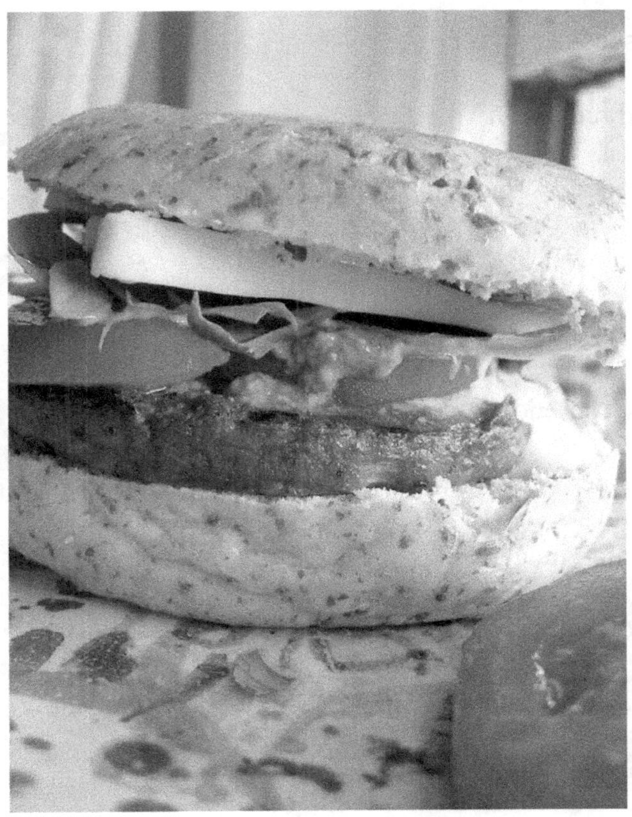

For many years, I use to be content just buying the frozen veggie burgers from my local grocery store. They are not bad, but they are not as good as this recipe will prove to you. You can use a few different things to prepare them; in this case, we propose using tofu as the main protein source. Let's do this!

Ingredients:

- 2 blocks of soft silk tofu

- 1 Tbsp. flax seeds

- 1 /4 cup diced red onion

- 2 cups chopped very finely fresh button mushrooms

- 1 tbsp. minced garlic

- 1 large egg

- 3 Tbsp. low fat shredded parmesan cheese

- Salt, black pepper

- 1 tbsp. balsamic vinegar

- 2 tbsp. olive oil

- Serve with sliced tomatoes or sliced cucumbers on the side

Servings: 4

Preparation time: 35-40 minutes

Nutritional information (per serving =1 patty)

Calories: 350

Carbs: 14g

Proteins: 17g

Fats: 9g

Method:

In a large bowl, place the well-drained tofu. Use a masher to mash them well and add the veggies, egg, flaxseeds and all other ingredients.

Form 4 large patties.

Heat some oil of your choice in a pan on medium heat and cook the 4 patties for about 5 minutes on each side.

Serve with toppings of your choice as suggested above.

Perfect cream of tomato soup

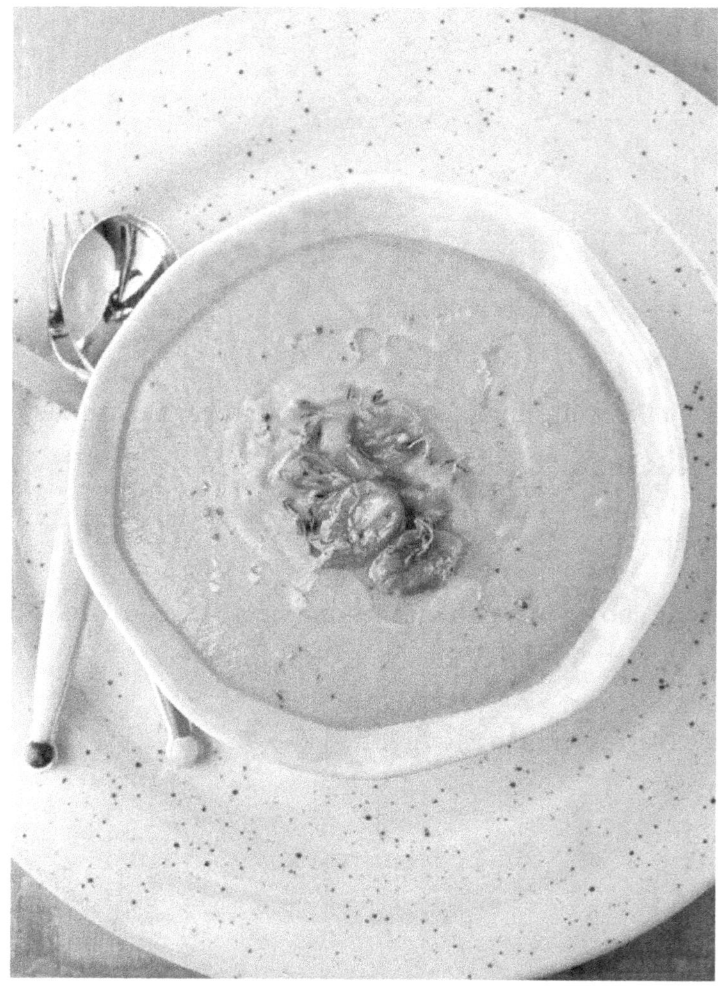

This homemade cream of tomato soup is very satisfying; if you ever had one before, you will be amazed by this recipe. Stop buying soups in cans, you never know exactly what they contain, and they usually are loaded with extra sodium and extra preservatives you really don't need in your healthy diet.

Ingredients:

- 1 small chopped onion

- 3 cups low fat turkey broth

- 2 tbsp. apple cider vinegar

- 1 large cooked sweet potato

- 1 Tbsp. minced garlic

- 6 large cooked fresh tomatoes

- 1 Tbsp. fresh minced basil

- Salt, black pepper

- 1 Tbsp. smoked paprika

- 3 cups skim milk

Servings: 4-6

Preparation time: 60 minutes

Nutritional information (per serving = 2 cups)

Calories: 175

Carbs: 19g

Proteins: 7g

Fats: 5g

Method:

Start by cooing the potato in the microwave on high temperature for about 4 minutes. It should be cooked enough that you can remove the flesh and place in the container of the high-speed blender.

In a medium pan, heat the oil and cook the diced fresh tomatoes with garlic basil and onion. Cook only 7-8 minutes at the most.

Add to the blender as well and add the rest of the ingredients listed above. You will probably have to blend in 2 batches as this might not all fit in your blender, depending on its size.

Activate the blender until the consistency is smooth

Place in a large saucepan and keep warm until it's time to serve.

Stuffed spinach and goat cheese chicken

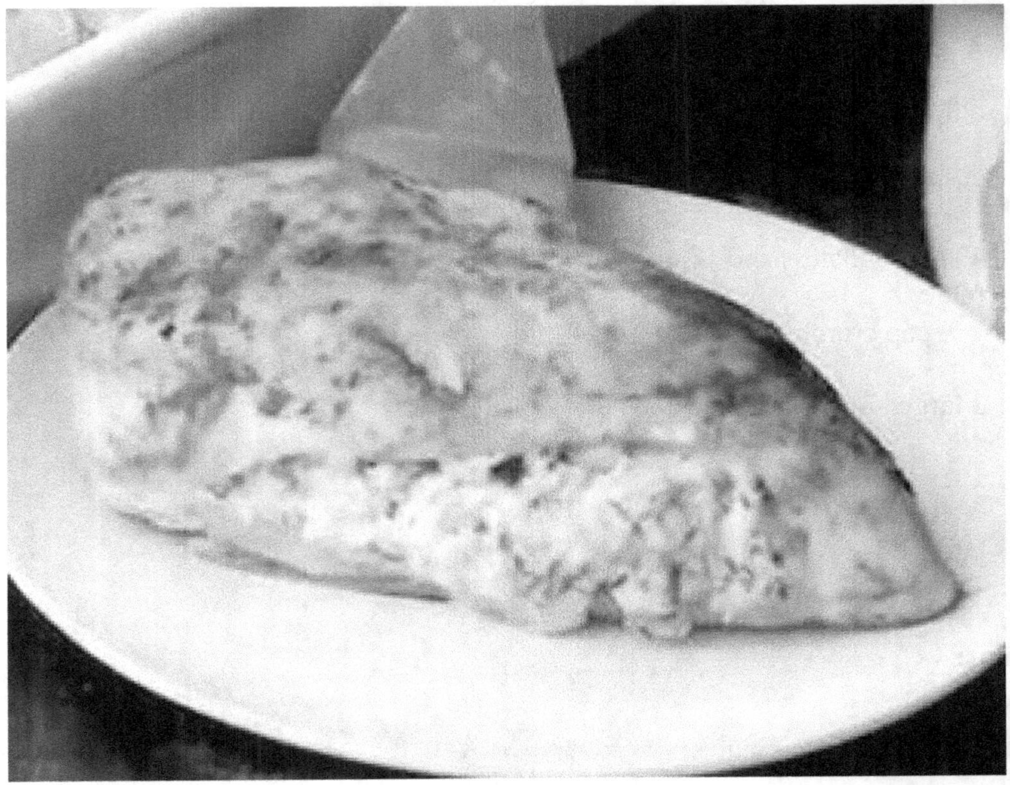

Because you are on a diet, you don't have to deprive yourself of all fancy meals. You can use a little fun and adventure, which is what this recipe is all about. Use fresh ingredients as always, please don't use frozen spinach, it might do the trick, but it loses so much flavor along the way.

Ingredients:

- 2 packages of fresh baby spinach leaves

- 3 Tbsp., minced garlic

- Salt, black pepper

- Dried cumin, about 1 Tbsp.

- 4 large boneless and skinless chicken breasts

- 1 ½ cup crumbled goat cheese

- 2 large lemon, for juice and zest

- 1 tbsp. Dijon mustard

- Olive oil

Servings: 4

Preparation time: 55 minutes

Nutritional information (per serving = 1 stuffed chicken breast)

Calories: 308

Carbs: 10g

Proteins: 30g

Fats: 15g

Method:

Preheat the oven to 375 degrees F.

Grease large baking dish and set aside.

Use a rolling pin to roll flat the chicken breast, after making an incision in each one. Season each of the breast with salt and pepper and set aside.

In a large saucepan heat oil and sautéed the spinach with garlic, seasonings, Dijon mustard and lemon juice. Cook for about 10 minutes.

Add the goat cheese quickly with the spinach and combine.

This will be the mixture you will use to stuff each chicken breast.

When folding the breast if it does not stay well, use a toothpick before placing in the oven for 45 minutes to cook.

Chickpea salad

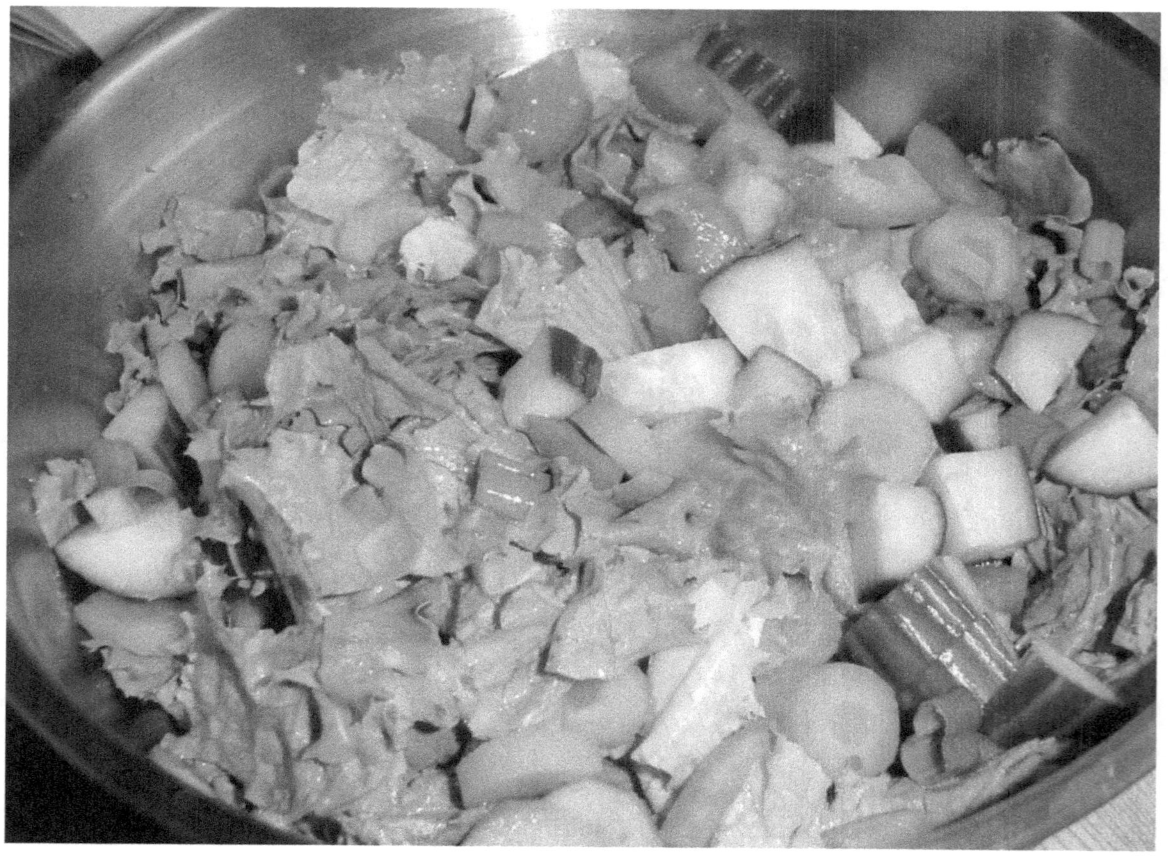

Now that you can reintroduce or introduce chickpeas into your diet, let's make this yummy salad together. This is the perfect dish to pack in your lunch or bring to a healthy work potluck. I learned that my kids love chickpeas, who knew! As always, make sure you only use fresh veggies and herbs.

Ingredients:

- 2 large cans chickpeas, well rinsed
- 2 minced green onions
- 1 tbsp. minced garlic
- 1 large diced red or orange bell pepper, your choice
- 2 Tbsp. olive oil
- ¼ cup sliced black olives
- ½ tsp onion salt
- Black pepper
- 1 Tbsp. fresh minced coriander
- Fresh minced parsley to decorate as ell

Servings: 4

Preparation time: 30 minutes

Nutritional information (per serving =1 cup)

Calories: 295

Carbs: 30g

Proteins: 11g

Fats: 65g

Method:

Use large mixing bowl or a storage container.

Dump the well rinsed and rinsed chickpeas. Add the onions, bell pepper, garlic and olives.

In a separate mixing bowl, combine the rest of the ingredients to make the dressing.

Pour onto the chickpeas and stir well.

Taste and adjust seasonings as needed.

Grilled corn and veggies side dish

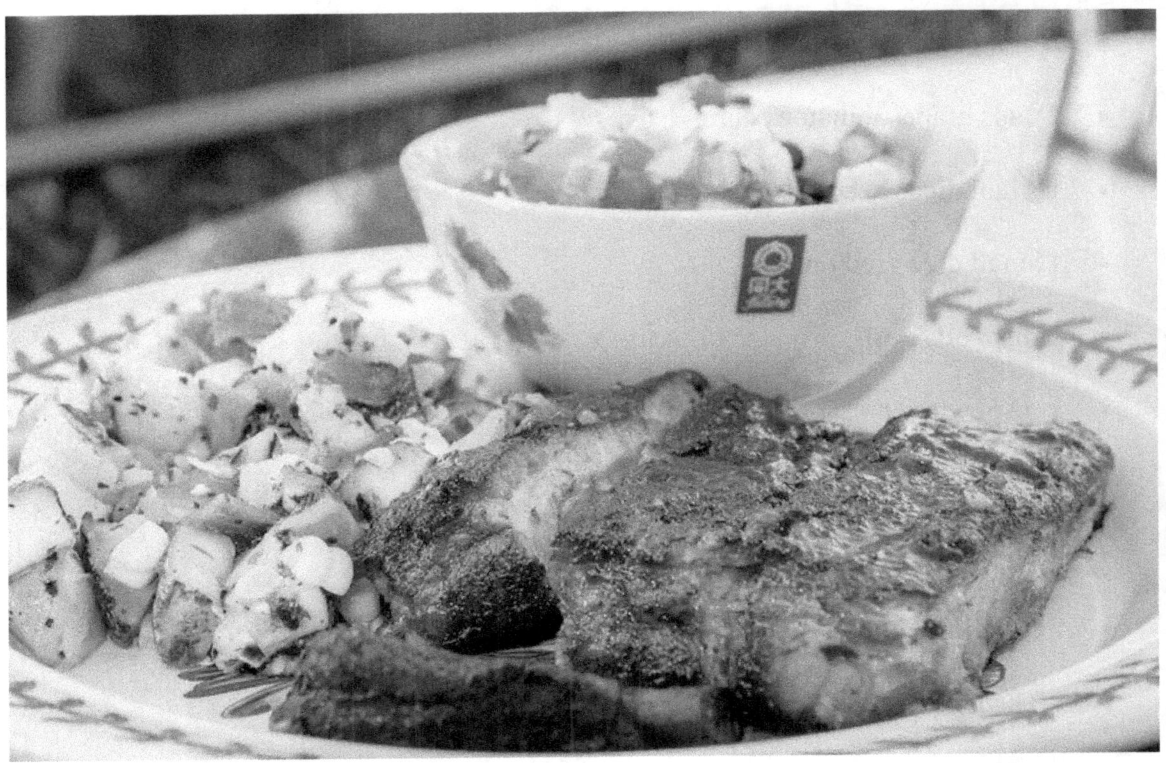

This will be one of the best eye-catching salads or side dishes you will ever create. The yellow, red, green, and other additional touches of color you will add make this dish simply irresistible. Now, you think it looks appetizing? Wait until you taste it, it is really yummy.

Ingredients:

- 1 large diced avocado

- 2 or 2 corn on the cob

- 2 cups grapes tomatoes cut in halves

- 1 small diced seedless cucumber

- 1 small diced red onion

- 2 tbsp. olive oil

- 1 tbsp. while balsamic vinegar

- ½ tsp. garlic powder

- Salt, pepper

- 2 tbsp. lime juice

- 1 Tbsp. taco seasonings.

Servings: 4-6

Preparation time: 40 minutes

Nutritional information (per serving = 1 cup)

Calories: 199

Carbs: 8g

Proteins: 8g

Fats: 9g

Method:

I usually make this side dish if I have left over corn on the cob I grilled the night before. I remove all the grains and place in a large salad bowl.

Then I add the rest of the veggies: tomatoes, onions, cucumber and avocados.

Add the lemon juice right way so the avocados do not turn black.

In a mixing bowl, combine the rest of the ingredients and then add to the colorful mixture.

Combine well and serve room temperature.

Low calorie lemon cake

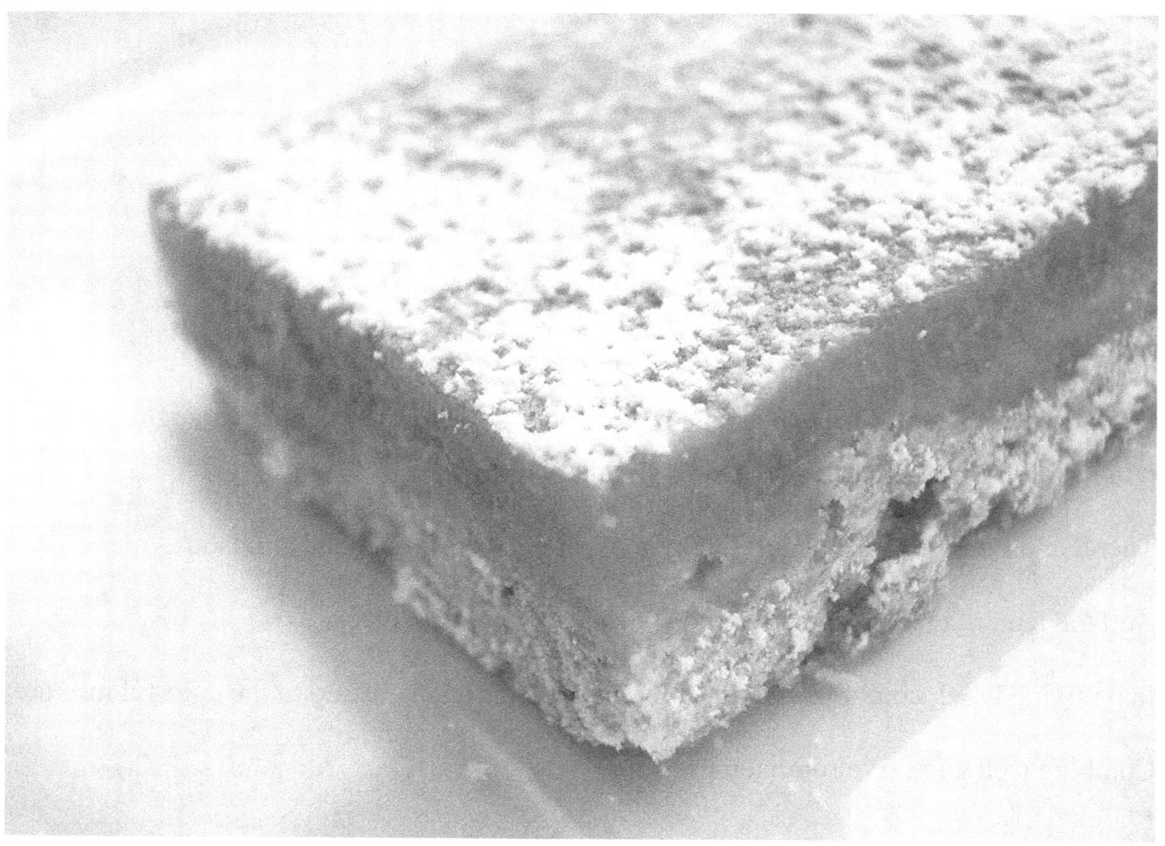

Have you always wondered if any diet would allow you to eat some cake? Now, I am not personally a fan of a big cake, but this is more like a snack cake type of treat, which is so light it is allowed on the south beach diet! So, this is a no brainer I bake this cake at least once a month, and we can enjoy it guilt-free as a family.

Ingredients:

- 1 1/2 cup almond flour

- 1 Tbs lemon extract

- 1 Tbsp. grated lemon zest

- ½ cup low fat sour cream

- ¾ cup coconut pam sugar

- 3 medium eggs

- 1/2 tsp. baking soda

- 1/2 tsp. baking powder

- 1/4 tsp. salt

- 1/3 cup coconut oil (room temperature)

Servings: 6-8

Preparation time: 50-55 minutes

Nutritional information (per serving = 1 slice)

Calories: 270

Carbs: 16g

Proteins: 22g

Fats: 15g

Method:

Preheat the oven to 350 degrees F.

Grease a cake pan and set aside.

In a large mixing bowl, combine the dry ingredients.

In a different bowl, combine the wet ingredients, starting by beating the eggs first. and then add on to each other.

Mix well so there are no lumps left.

Pour into the cake dish and bake for 50 minutes.

Low carbs spaghetti meatballs

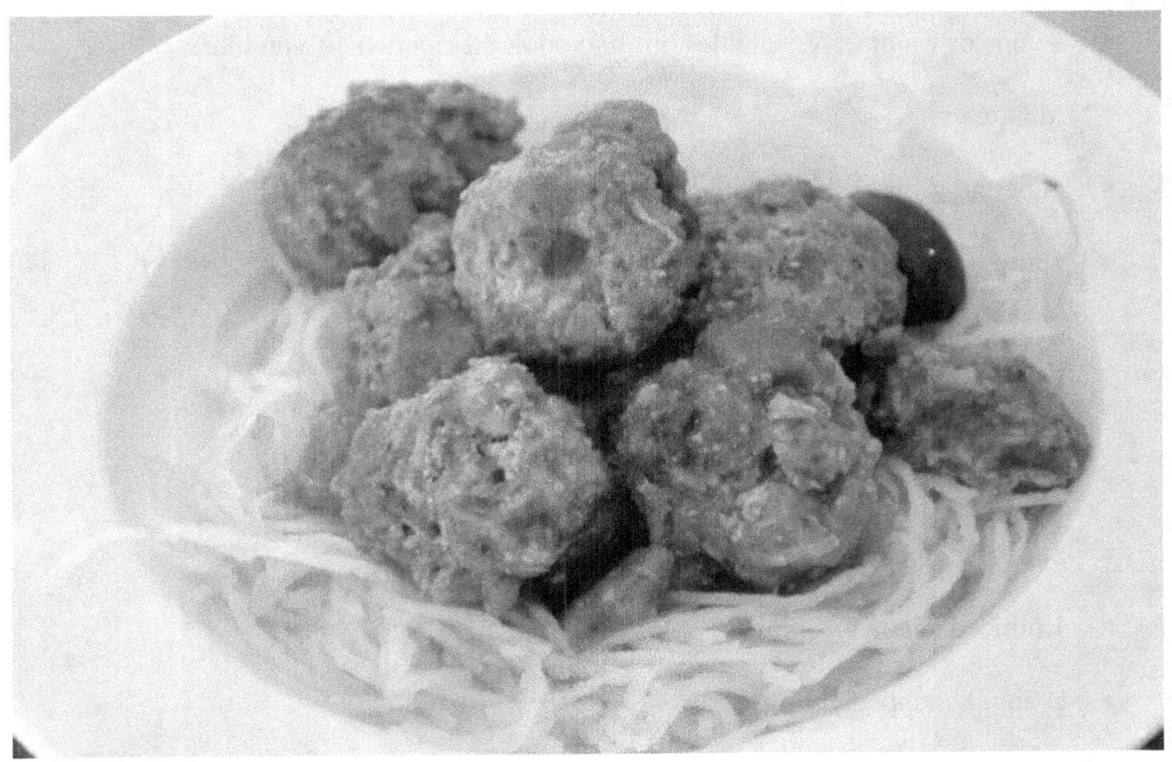

Because you are not allowed to eat pasta and grains in the first phase of your diet, it does not mean that they are forbidden forever. They are many great options to keep it gluten free or low carb. We love to use buckwheat noodles in our household, they have a unique taste, and they are super nutritious. Also, of course, the meatballs are made from scratch with chicken ground meat.

Ingredients:

- 1 bag or ½ pound buckwheat noodles

- 4 cups or water or Vegetables broth to cook the noodles, if you like

- Meatballs

- ¾ pound ground chicken meat

- 1 large egg

- 2 tbsp. flaxseeds

- 6 Tbsp. parmesan cheese

- 1 Tbsp. Italian seasonings

- Salt, black pepper

- 1 minced small zucchini

- ½ small chopped yellow onion

- 1 tbsp. minced garlic

- 2 tbsp. olive oil + more when serving the noodles

- ¼ cup fresh mixed herbs: basil oregano, parsley and chives

Servings: 4-6

Preparation time: 60 minutes

Nutritional information (per serving = 1 cup noodles 1 cup of stir fry)

Calories: 320

Carbs: 22g

 Proteins: 22g

Fats: 20g

Method:

Preheat your oven to 400 degrees F.

Grease a large baking sheet and then set aside.,

In a large mixing bowl, mix the ingredients for the meatballs with your hands.

Form small meatballs and place them to cook o the baking sheet for about 40 minutes.

Meanwhile, make the buckwheat noodles, suing the broth to give more flavor.

When the meatballs are done, add a little olive oil to the noodles with fresh herbs and serve with the meatballs on top.

Refreshing alcohol free mojitos

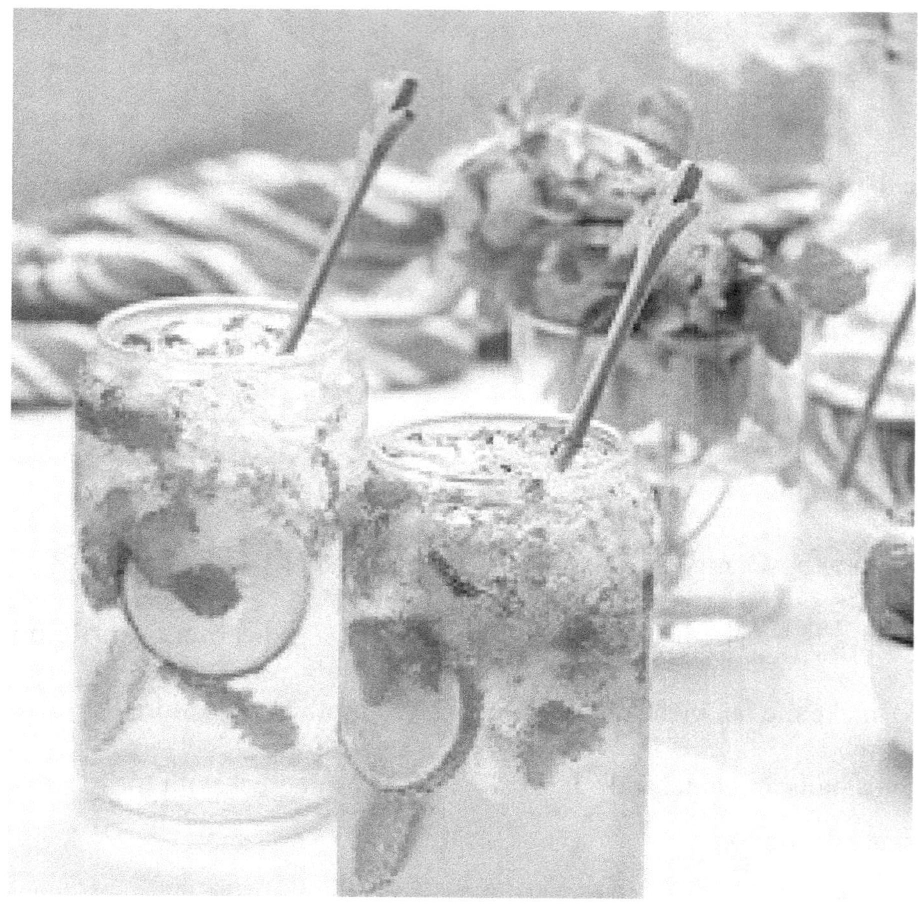

If you are going to make mojitos, you need to use fresh mint leaves. Well, although we will not use any alcohol to keep our version of the mojitos low in calories, don't worry, we will use plenty of mints. Get ready for probably what will become your favorite drink of the summer!

Ingredients:

- ¼ cup fresh mint leaves

- 2 Tbsp. agave syrup

- 1 cup 100% juice, no sugar added of cherry juice

- 1 cup 100% juice, no sugar added cranberry juice

- 2 Tbsp. lime juice

- 2 cups ice cubes

Servings: 4-6

Preparation time: 30-60 minutes

Nutritional information (per serving =1 glass)

Calories: 178

Carbs: 13g

Proteins: 4 g

Fats: 1g

Method:

I suggest you use a pitcher and mix all the ingredients and let the mint leaves soak a little while.

But if you are in a hurry just divide up the ingredients and make a glass at a time.

Healthy grilled chicken skewers

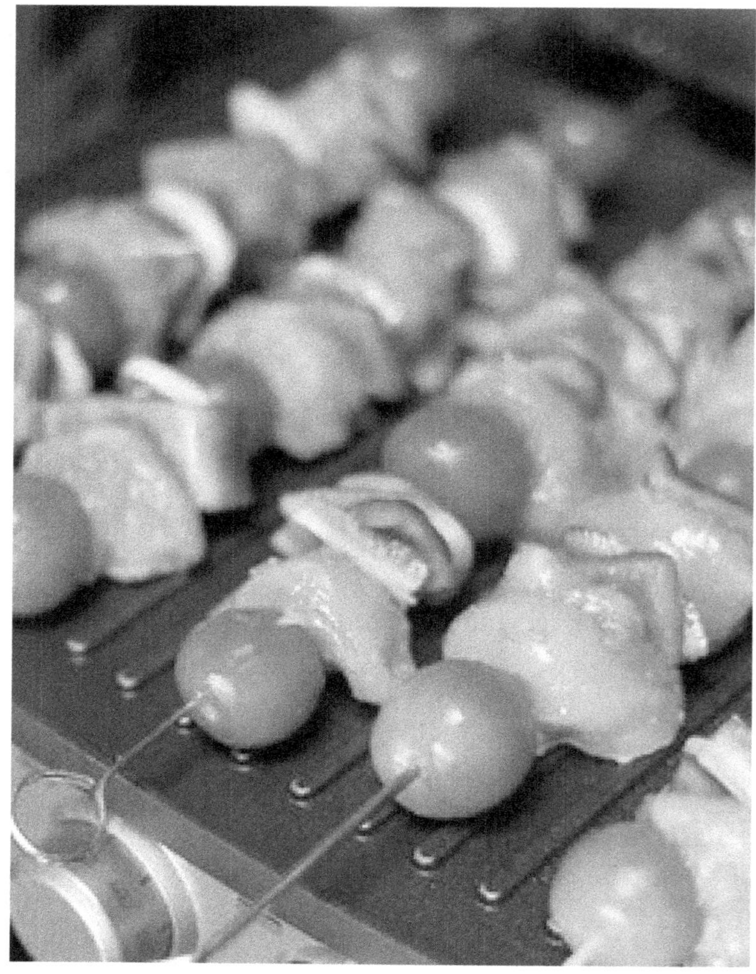

Light up your grills! Summer has arrived, and so have the delicious ways to cook and serve chicken. It will be better to plan ahead and marinate the chicken in our special low-calorie mix, and then you are ready to cook these delicious skewers in no time, any night of the week!

Ingredients:

- ½ pound chicken breast, boneless and skinless, cut in large chunks
- 1 large green pepper cut in chunks
- 1 large zucchini cut in chunks
- 1 medium red onion cut in chunks
- About 12-16 grapes tomatoes

Marinade

- 3 tbsp. sesame oil
- 2 tbsp. rice wine
- 1 tbsp. fresh minced ginger
- 1 tbsp. minced garlic
- 1 Tbsp. cayenne pepper
- Salt, black pepper
- Skewers

Servings: 4

Preparation time: 45 minutes + marinating time

Nutritional information (per serving =)

Calories: 279

Carbs: 16g

Proteins: 27g

Fats: 14g

Method:

In a bowl, combine the ingredients for the marinade and try to marinade the chicken cubes for at least an hour ahead.

Start up the grill or you could very cook at 400 dress f in the oven if you wish, you think the chicken has marinated enough.

Prepare all the veggies and use poke away a combination of chicken and veggie son each skewer.

Use a brush to also add a little marinade on the veggies.

Grill for about 15 minutes total.

Serve right way.

Wheat pita toast with mango and mahi-mahi

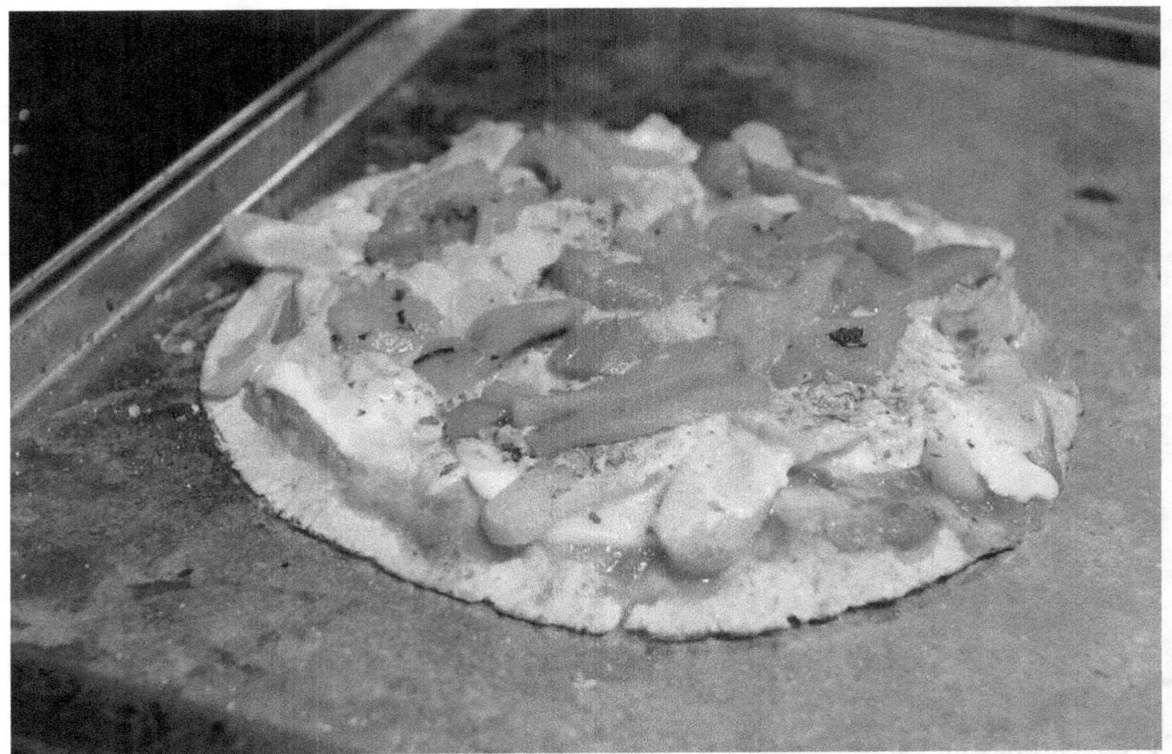

As you know by now, this is not allowed in the first phase of your diet, but it can be introduced in the second one. Mahi mahi is a nice flaky white fish, and it marries well with fresh mango. I like to add some cilantro and other spices, of course, as it can taste very plain fish if you don't season it well.

Ingredients:

- 2 or 3 mahi mahi filets

- 4-8 pita wheat bread, depending on size

- 2 tbsp. olive oil

- Salt, black pepper

- 2 tbsp. fresh minced cilantro

- 1 medium mango peeled and diced

- 1 Tbsp. lemon juice

- ½ tsp cumin

- Serve with lemon wedges as well

Servings: 4

Preparation time: 40-45 minutes

Nutritional information (per serving =)

Calories: 233

Carbs: 18g

Proteins: 22g

Fats: 75g

Method:

Preheat the oven to 400 degrees F.

Grease a large baking sheet.

Cut the pita bread in halves with a kike. Place on the baking sheet.

In a bowl, combine the diced mango, lemon juice, cumin, cilantro, oil. Set aside.

In a medium frying pan fry the fish after seasonings with salt and pepper only for about 15 minutes.

Place the pita bread sin the oven so they get toasted.

Remove the bread form oven and place pieces of fish and a generous portion of the mango mixture on top of each pita bread.

Delightful stuffed crepes

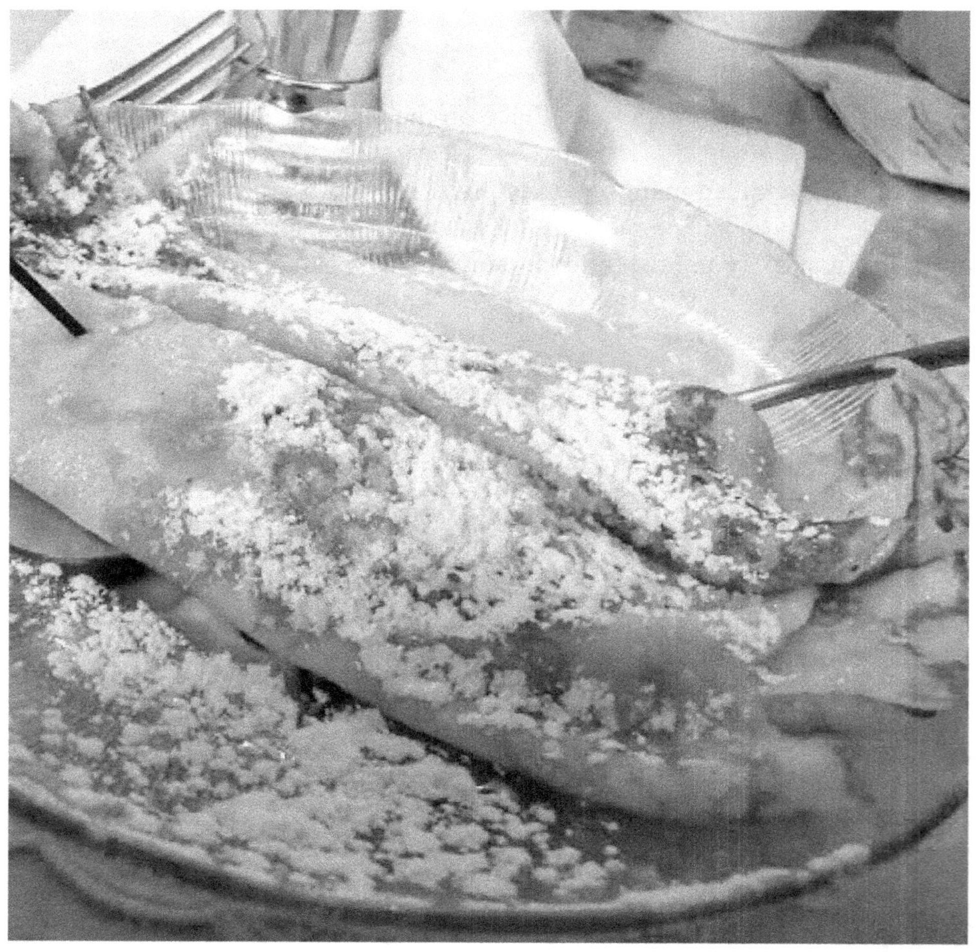

Let's finish with this beautiful and original recipe. Let's stuff some.

Ingredients:

- 1/3 cup coconut flour

- 2 Tbsp. chia seeds

- ½ tsp. salt

- ¼ cup coconut unsweetened milk

- 1 large egg

- 4 Tbsp. coconut oil (room temperature)

Filling:

- 1 cup low fat cottage cheese

- 2 cups favorite berries: blueberries, strawberries, blackberries raspberries if they

  are fresh, your choice

- 4 Tbsp. maple syrup

Servings: 4

Preparation time: 35-40 minutes

Nutritional information (per serving =1 crepe with about 2 tbsp. cheese, ¼ cup fruits and some maple syrup)

Calories: 230

Carbs: 29g

Proteins: 22g

Fats: 8g

Method:

Let's start making the crepes mixture. In a medium bowl, combine all dry ingredients.

Add the coconut oil, milk and egg and mix well.

Use addental coconut oil t heat in a pan and start making the crepes one by one.

Plate one crepe per person with a little cottage cheese, some fresh fruits and a tablespoon of maple syrup.

This is a meal for the phase 3 of the south beach diet.

Fresh kale and tuna salad

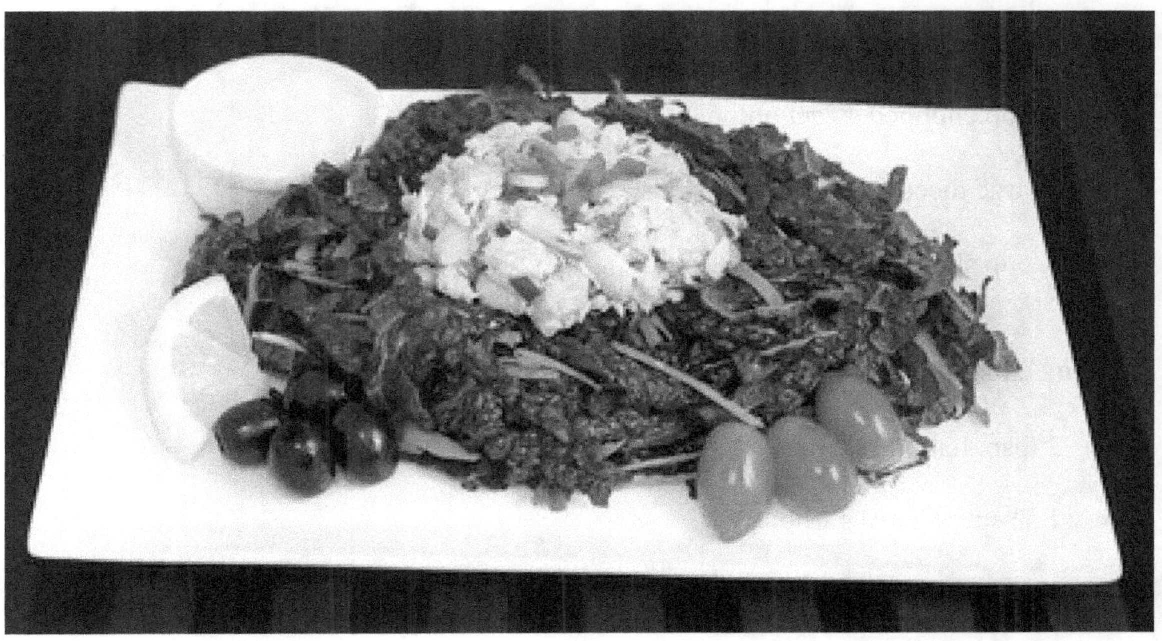

Now, only this salad simply screams freshness, but it will taste amazing if you follow the simple steps below. Make sure you buy some very fresh kale and rinse it off thoroughly as it may still contain some soil residue. Kale can be slightly bitter but don't worry, the other ingredients we add in the salad will balance it out nicely.

Ingredients:

- 1 large package of fresh kale

- 2 large cans whiter tuna, well drained (in olive oil is fine)

- ½ cup chopped sweet onion

- 2 large diced grapevine tomatoes

- ¼ cup sliced green olives

Dressing

- 2 tbsp. lemon juice

- 1 Tbsp. Minced garlic

- 1 tbsp. Dijon mustard

- Salt, black

- 4 Tbsp. olive oil

Servings: 4-6

Preparation time: 30-60 minutes

Nutritional information (per serving =)

Calories: 196

Carbs: 11g

Proteins: 19g

Fats: 13g

Method:

In a small mixing bowl, combine the ingredients for the dressing and set aside.

Plate the salad with generous portion of fresh kale, ¼ of the tuna meat, and all the other veggies listed.

Add some dressing and you are all set!

Ridiculously easy cabbage soup

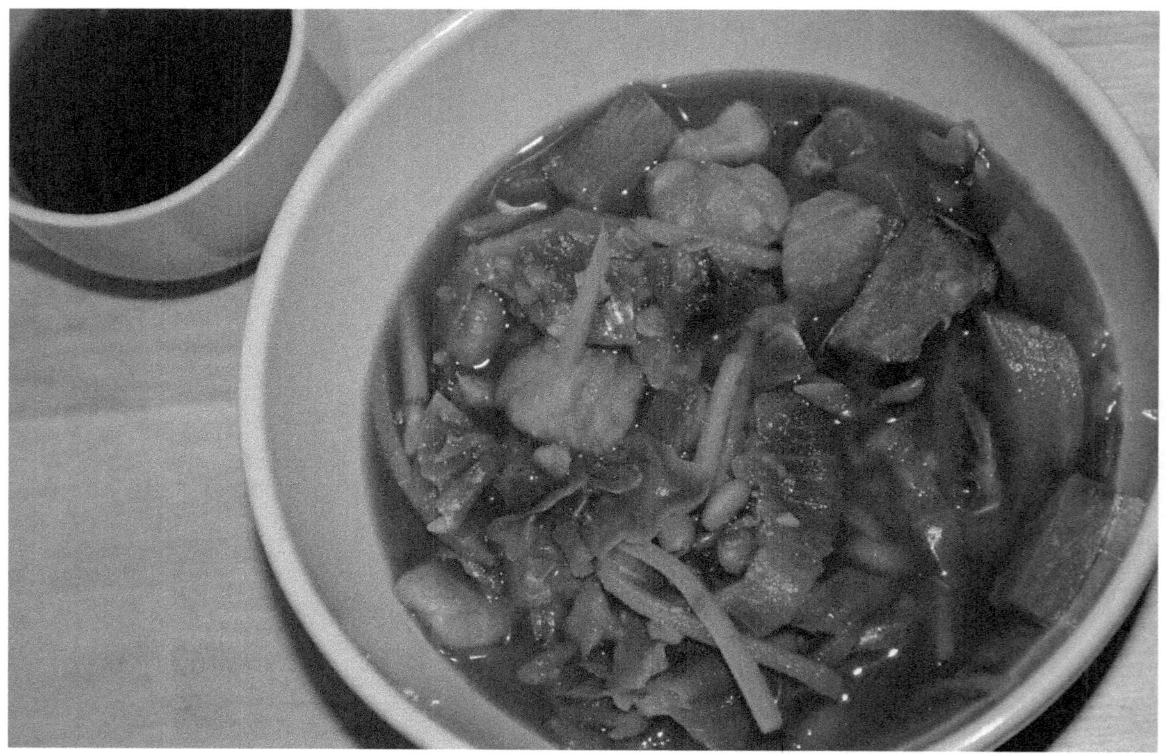

You can use a large pot on the stovetop or your slow cooker to make this easy recipe. Either way, it is going to turn out just yummy and healthy as expected.

Ingredients:

- 6 cups fresh chopped green cabbage

- 6 cups vegetables broth

- 2 mediums size carrots peeled and chopped

- 4 cups spinach

- 2 medium chopped yellow onions

- 2 tbsp. minced garlic

- 1 Tbsp. Italian. seasonings

- ¼ cup fresh minced parsley

- 2 tbsp. lemon juice

- 1 large can dice tomatoes with chilies

- Salt, black pepper

- 1 Tbsp. cayenne pepper

Servings: 4-6

Preparation time: 60 minutes+

Nutritional information (per serving =2 cups)

Calories: 310

Carbs: 16g

Proteins: 17g

Fats: 10g

Method:

Use a large pot and heat some olive oil and cook the onions, garlic, green cabbage and sliced carrots for about 10 minutes.

Add the broth next with the canned tomatoes and all the seasonings.

Let the soup simmer for about 50 minutes or so and serve warm.

If you use the slow cooker, cook on low temperature for about 4-5 hours.

Super yummy chocolate muffins

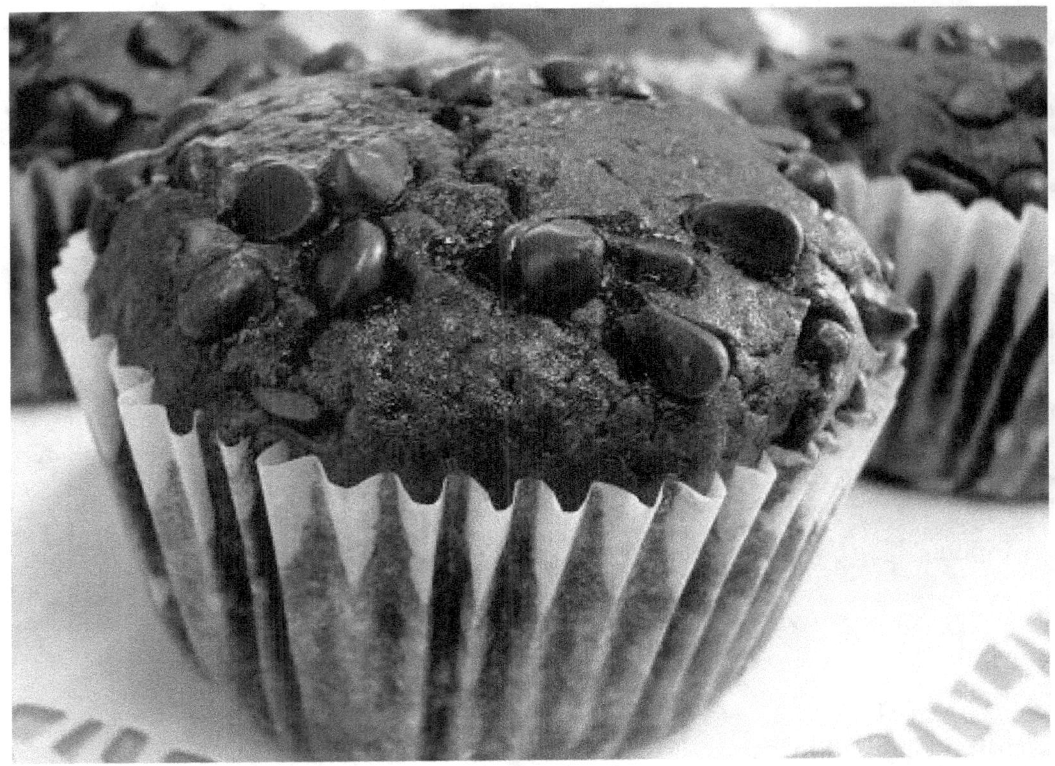

If you knew you could eat chocolate muffins while being on a diet, perhaps you would have started dieting earlier, right? You will understand why it is important to follow this recipe. You don't want to add unwanted fats or the wrong type of flour because your calories and carb count will go up considerably.

Ingredients:

- ½ cup almond butter

- 2 eggs

- ¼ cup low fat ricotta cheese

- 3 tbsp. cocoa powder

- 1 tbsp. instant coffee of your choice

- 3 Tbsp. agave syrup

- 1 /2 baking powder

- ½ tsp. baking soda

- Pinch salt

Servings: 6-8

Preparation time: 50 minutes

Nutritional information (per serving =1 muffin)

Calories: 325

Carbs: 29g

 Proteins: 17g

Fats: 15g

Method:

Preheat the oven to 350 degrees F.

Get a muffin tin out with 8 muffin papers and spray lightly with cooking spray.

In a first mixing bowl, combine the dry ingredients.

Add gradually the eggs, ricotta cheese, almond butter and agave syrup.

Combine until the consistency is perfect.

Pour into the baking dish and bake for 35-40-minutes or until done.

Simple eggplant parmesan

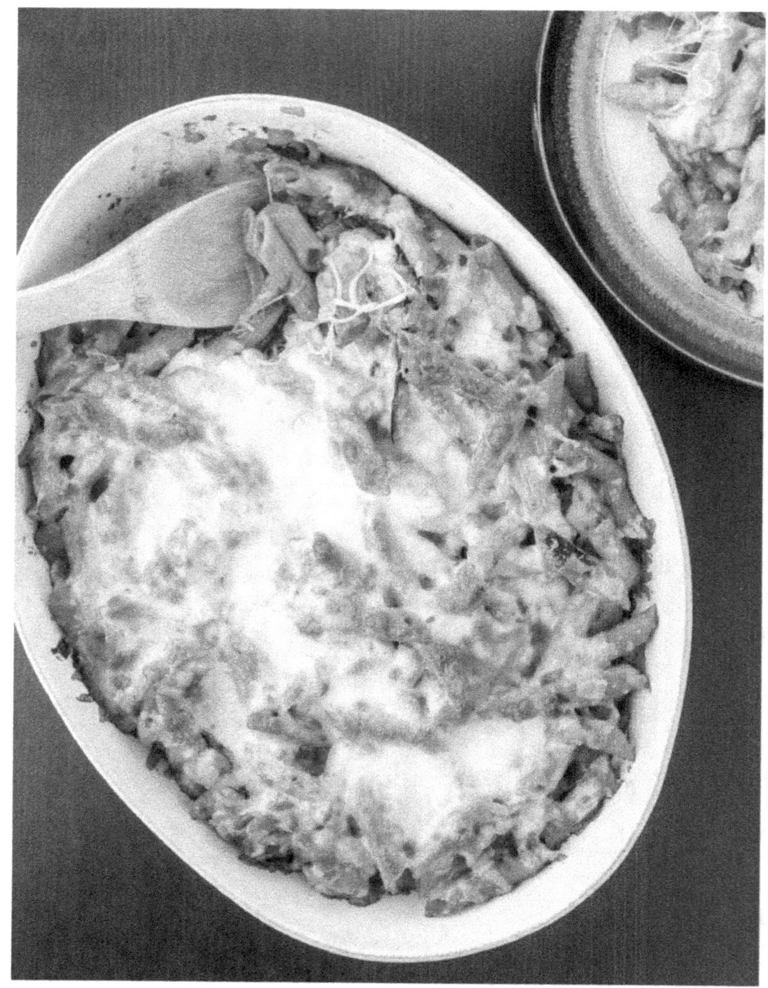

This recipe will make you think you are out in a fancy Italian restaurant. Use the right sauce, cheese and spices, and all will be well. Also, make sure you cook the eggplant just right as we will indicate below.

Ingredients:

- 2 large eggplant cut lengthwise

- 3 tbsp. olive oil

- 1 cup low fat shredded Mozzarella cheese

- 2 cups tomatoes sauce, your favorite if natural, it can be homemade, but it does not have to be

- 2 cups crumbled feta cheese

- 1 Tbsp. fresh minced basil

- 1 tbsp. dried Italian seasoning

- Salt, black pepper

Servings: 4

Preparation time: 60 minutes

Nutritional information (per serving =)

Calories: 378

Carbs: 16g

Proteins: 22g

Fats: 15g

Method:

Preheat oven to 450°F.

In a baking dish, place all pieces of eggplant (4) cut lengthwise prior.

Brush each eggplant with olive oil and season with pepper and salt.

Bake in the oven for about 40 minutes.

Remove from the oven then turn the eggplant ver. Topped them off with the tomato sauce and a layer of mozzarella cheese and finish the off with crumbled feta cheese.

Sprinkle the Italian seasonings and fresh basil.

Put back I the oven for 20-25 minutes until eh cheese is perfectly melted.

Corn and greens veg sandwich

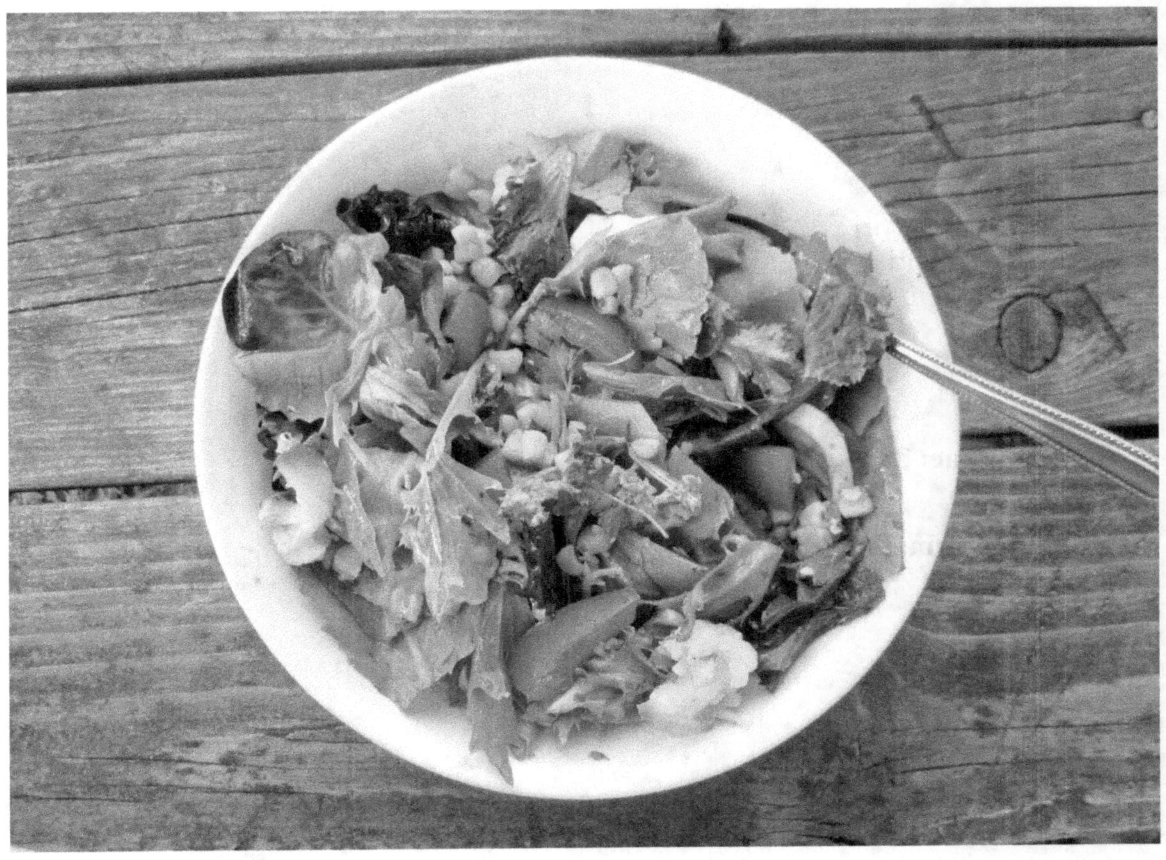

Who needs crackers to make some awesome appetizers? Let's use sliced cucumber and add some fresh smoked salmon, capers, and all will be well in the low carb's world.

Ingredients:

- 1 or 2 seedless English cucumber

- ½ pound smoked salmon slices

- 3 Tbsp. capers

- 1 lemon

- Smoked paprika

Servings: 10-24

Preparation time: 20 minutes

Nutritional information (per serving = 2 bites = 140)

Calories: 140

Carbs: 12g

Proteins: 22g

Fats: 13g

Method:

Use a large serving plate.

Slice the cucumbers about ½ inch thick.

Cut he smoked salmon in small ices to fit a cucumber slice and apply on top followed by a few capers.

Sprinkle a little paprika on top for color and taste.

Then squeeze just enough lemon juice to make it worth!

Soft and tasty corn bread

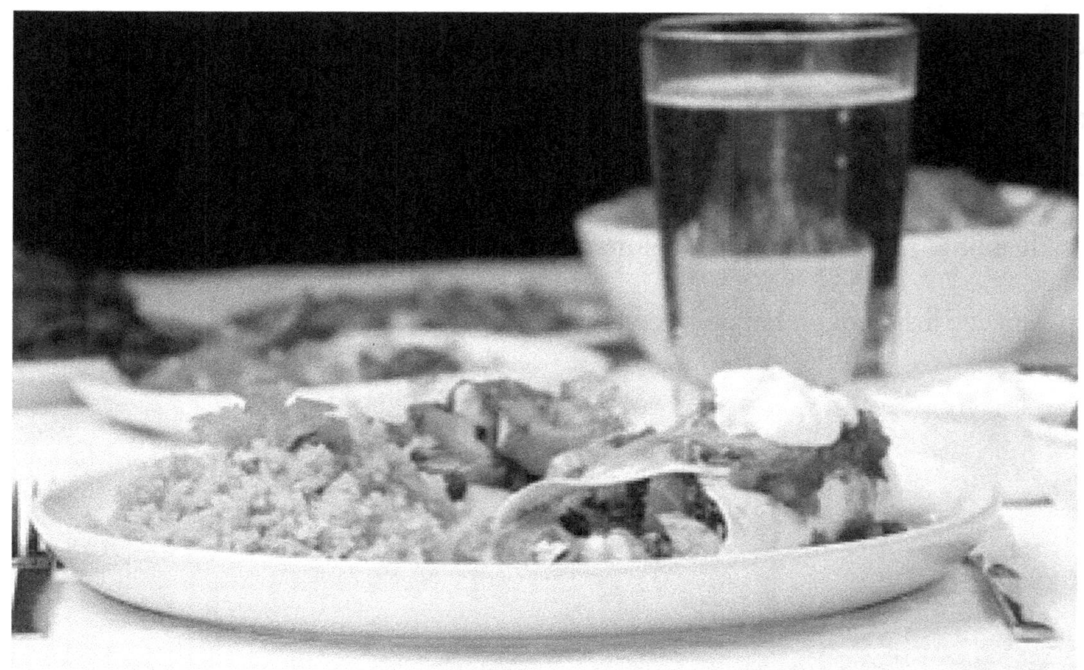

No need to explain how truly awesome zucchinis noodles are as a replacement for carb loaded pasta or rice. They are not only healthy but look so pretty on your plate. Let's make a very simple and delicious dish right now.

Ingredients:

- 4 cups zucchini noodles

- 1 cup cherry tomatoes

- 3 tablespoons sliced green stuffed with pimentos olives

- ½ cup shredded Parmesan cheese

- Olive oil

- 1 tbsp. Balsamic vinegar

- 1 tbsp. minced fresh parsley

- 1 tbsp. mince fresh basil

- Salt, pepper

Servings: 3-4

Preparation time: 30 minutes

Nutritional information (per serving =2 cups)

Calories: 210

Carbs: 17g

Proteins: 17g

Fats: 11g

Method:

Use the mandolin to make the zucchini noodles and prepare all together ingredients head as well.

In a large frying pan heat oil and fry the onions,

I usually like to steam the zucchini noodles for just a few before sautéed them as well in the frying pan. Drain well and fry for 10 minutes with the rest of the ingredients, except the cheese.

Sprinkle the parmesan cheese as you are serving.

Salmon casserole

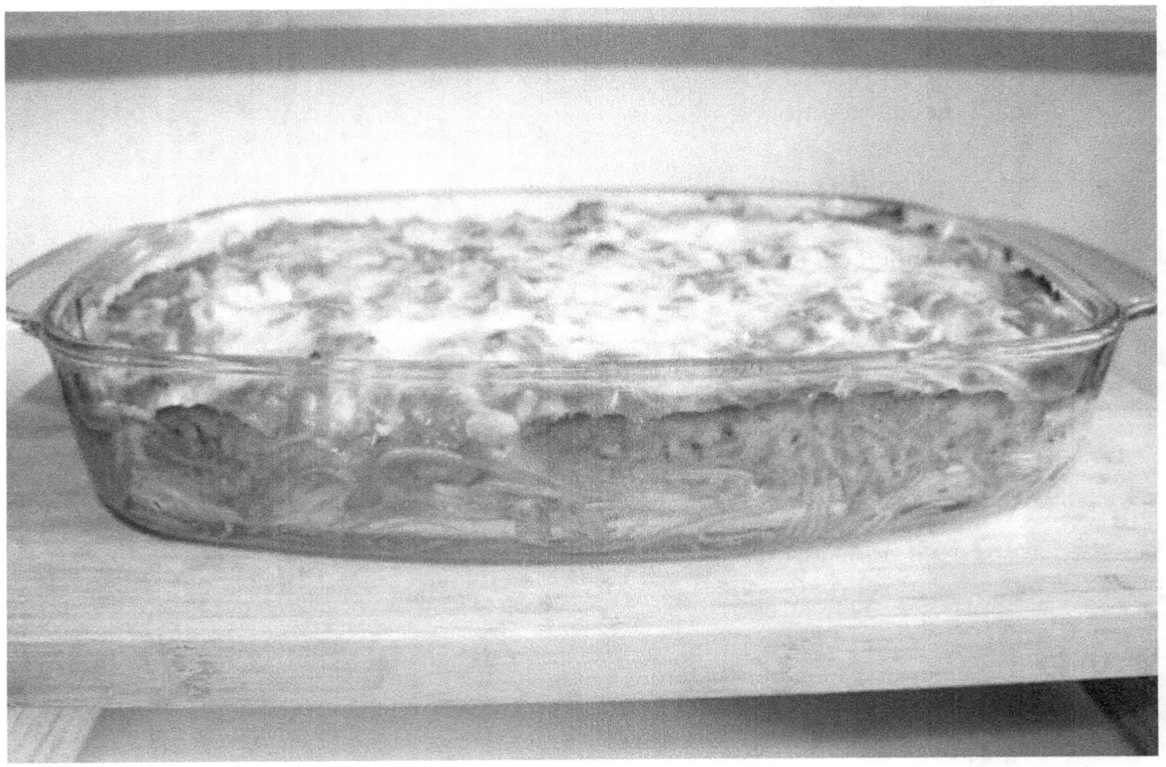

Let's finish with this beautiful and original recipe. Let's stuff some.

Ingredients:

- 4 cups cooked green beans
- 2 large can canned salmon, well drained
- 1 small diced red onion
- 4 large hardboiled eggs
- 3 large chopped celery stalks
- 3 tbsp. olive oil
- Salt, black pepper
- ½ tsp. dry mustard
- 1 tbsp. fresh minced chives

Servings: 4-6

Preparation time: 55-60 minutes

Nutritional information (per serving =)

Calories: 325

Carbs: 17g

Proteins: 29g

Fats: 19g

Method:

In a large mixing bowl, combine the cooked green beans, onions and celery with the oil with all seasoning and herbs.

Mix well. Cut in small pieces the hardboiled eggs and add next.

Finally, after draining well, add the salmon meat and the onion, celery.

Combine again and serve on 4 different plates.

Season again with more pepper if needed.

Mashed cauliflower

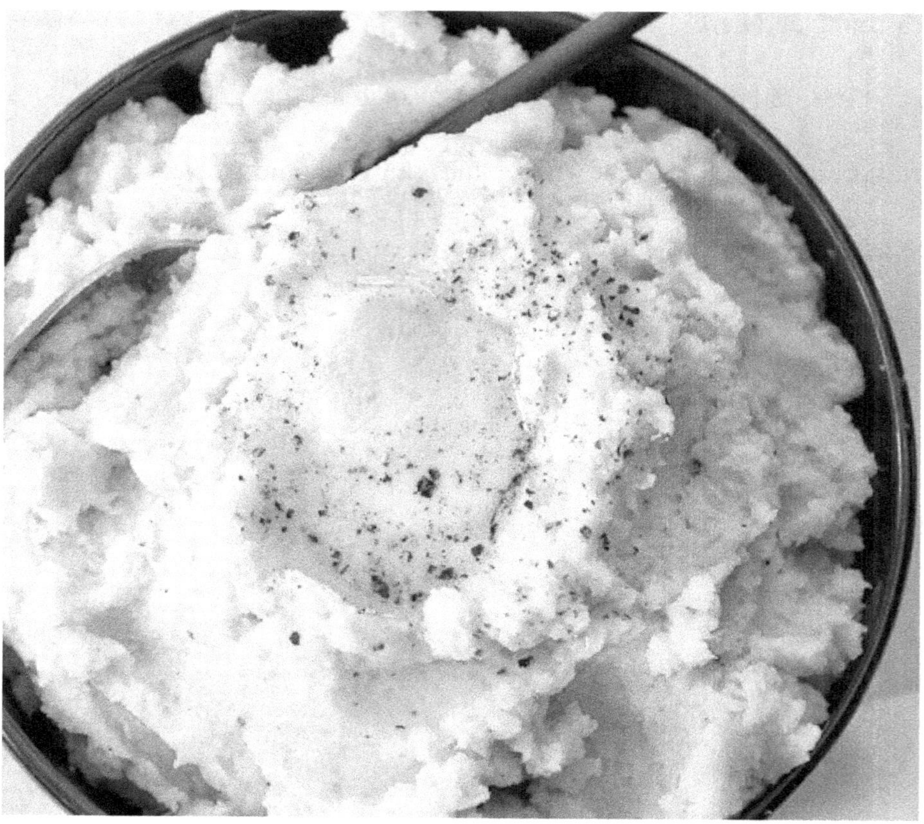

This side dish is the perfect replacement for mashed potato casserole. Soon enough, even your kids will end up requesting it!

Ingredients:

- 1 large cauliflower head

- 2 cups 2 % milk

- ½ tsp. garlic powder

- ½ tsp. onion powder

- 2 Tbsp. minced fresh parsley

- Salt, white pepper

- 4 tbsp. gee butter

Servings: 4-6

Preparation time: 40 minutes

Nutritional information (per serving =)

Calories: 179

Carbs: 12g

Proteins: 12g

Fats: 6g

Method:

Boil water in a large pot and using s trainer, steam cook your broccoli head, you previously cut in small pieces.

When it's done, add into a large mixing bowl with the milk, the butter, spices and herbs.

Use the electric mixer to reduce into a nice smooth puree.

Serve way!

Conclusion

Because we could not give you all the answers in the introduction of this cookbook, we would love to add some valuable information here on a diet itself and the related health concerns. So, let's basically answer some random questions about the diet we anticipated you might have.

Random south beach diet questions

Why is the south beach diet known as efficient?

Because this diet is telling you to cut out carbs or keep them very low, you will automatically help manage your blood sugar levels more efficiently. So, by doing so, your insulin levels will be stabilized. In the scheme of things, this will also mean that because you give your body less sugar and starchy foods, the less your bloodstream will have to absorb them, and the less fat or weight you will gain, just by that simple concept.

South beach diet vs. Atkins diet, is there really a difference between the 2 dieting tools?

The answer is yes. They are named differently, so they very unalike. Here are some highlights. Atkins is a diet regarding when it comes to the quantity of carbs you can eat. The south beach diet is trying to teach you to be picky about the carbs you will eat and reintroduce good food in your life. Now, don't get us wrong, they are similar diets, but if you explore them in detail you will quickly know the difference. One might be better than another for certain individuals with specific health concerns, and again, we recommend for you to seek your primary care physician.

Let's review pros and cons of the diet

The south beach diet is relatively easy to follow. You do not have to weigh your food or count the calories you eat every day. You can eventually have a variety of foods, so the frustration or hunger is kept to a minimum. However, keep in mind like any other diet; you should take extra time to prepare the foods you used to prepare, removing the carbs. Also, during the first phase, you might feel a little frustrated, which is very understandable.

You will lose some weight, especially in the first phase, and will create some awesome lifestyle and dieting habits for life. You can snack or eat several little meals a day, however, you must carefully choose the food you eat.

Although, like any other diet, the south beach diet might not be appropriate for everyone, it can certainly help many people improve their health conditions considerably. You need to make sure you have enough nutrients, according to your age group.

It is a diet that can easily be followed if you are eating out at restaurants or at your work cafeteria. Make sure you are requesting your server to make some small changes to your order, such as removing the rice, potatoes, or breads form your meal before serving.

We wish you all the best in your journey to a lighter and healthier you. As always, it was our pleasure to share with you the most amazing recipes we like to make at home and hopefully, many tips that will last you for a lifetime.

Author's Afterthoughts

Thanks ever so much to each of my cherished readers for investing the time to read this book!

I know you could have picked from many other books, but you chose this one. So, a big thanks for downloading this book and reading all the way to the end.

If you enjoyed this book or received value from it, I'd like to ask you for a favor. Please take a few minutes to post an honest and heartfelt review on Amazon.com. Your support does make a difference and helps to benefit other people.

Thanks for your Reviews!

Rachael Rayner